—— Second Edition ——

DOCUMENTATION STRATEGIES TO SUPPORT SEVERITY OF ILLNESS

Ensure an Accurate Professional Profile

Robert S. Gold, MD

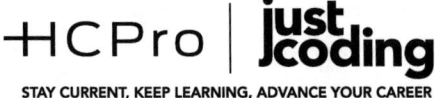

STAY CURRENT, KEEP LEARNING, ADVANCE YOUR CAREER

Documentation Strategies to Support Severity of Illness: Ensure an Accurate Professional Profile, Second Edition, is published by HCPro, Inc.

Copyright © 2011 HCPro, Inc.

Cover Image © VikaSuh. Used under license from Shutterstock.com.

All rights reserved. Printed in the United States of America.   5   4   3   2   1

ISBN: 978-1-60146-859-8

No part of this publication may be reproduced, in any form or by any means, without prior written consent of HCPro, Inc., or the Copyright Clearance Center (978/750-8400). Please notify us immediately if you have received an unauthorized copy.

HCPro, Inc., provides information resources for the healthcare industry.

HCPro, Inc., is not affiliated in any way with The Joint Commission, which owns the JCAHO and Joint Commission trademarks.

Robert S. Gold, MD, Author
Janet L. Morris, Senior Managing Editor
Ilene MacDonald, Executive Editor
Lauren McLeod, Editorial Director
Karin Holmes, Proofreader

Mike Mirabello, Senior Graphic Artist
Matt Sharpe, Production Manager
Shane Katz, Art Director
Jean St. Pierre, Senior Director of Operations

Advice given is general. Readers should consult professional counsel for specific legal, ethical, or clinical questions. Arrangements can be made for quantity discounts. For more information, contact:

HCPro, Inc.
75 Sylvan Street, Suite A-101
Danvers, MA 01923
Telephone: 800/650-6787 or 781/639-1872
Fax: 800/639-8511
E-mail: *customerservice@hcpro.com*

To order more copies of this handbook, visit HCPro online at
***www.hcmarketplace.com* or call customer service at 800/650-6787.**

08/2011
21903

Contents

About the Author v

Introduction 1

Acute Myocardial Infarction 3

Adverse Effects of Medications 6

Alcohol/Substance Use/Abuse 9

Anemia 10

Chest Pain/Angina 14

Chronic Obstructive Pulmonary Disease 17

Comfort Measures Only 19

Comorbidities (Comorbid Conditions) 21

Complications (Postoperative) 22

Coronary Artery Disease 25

Debridement 27

Dementia/Delirium/Encephalopathy 29

Femur Fracture—Treatment 34

Gastrointestinal Bleed 37

Heart Failure 39

Hyperglycemia 44

Low Anterior Resection 46

Malignancies 48

Malnutrition 50

Obesity 54

Pneumonia 57

Pulmonary Edema 60

Renal Failure 62

Respiratory Failure 65

Seizures 68

Sepsis 71

Stroke/Cerebrovascular Accident 73

Symptoms 77

Syncope 78

Trauma 80

About the Author

Robert S. Gold, MD

Robert S. Gold, MD, has more than 40 years of experience as a physician, medical director, and consultant. A graduate of Hahnemann Medical College in Philadelphia, he trained in general surgery in the U.S. Navy, where he spent his professional career as a practicing surgeon.

Since leaving the service, he has worked as a consultant in the fields of managed care medicine, locum tenens, home health, hospital accreditation and licensure, and, most notably during the past 16 years, in audit and education regarding documentation, coding, and billing accuracy for healthcare services.

Dr. Gold is known nationally for his educational presentations regarding the clinical orientation of coding in American Health Information Management Association and HCPro audio conferences. He has spoken at national and state-level Health Information Management and Association of Clinical Documentation Improvement Specialists meetings about the participation of the medical staff in programs of documentation improvement. He writes the monthly columns *Clinically Speaking* for **Briefings on Coding Compliance Strategies** and *Minute for the Medical Staff* for **Medical Records Briefing.**

Dr. Gold also is a cofounder of DCBA, Inc., a consulting company that provides physician-led programs in clinical documentation improvement, along with coder education in the diagnoses and procedures to which they assign codes. His programs lead to increased compliance, appropriate reflection of true severity of illness, and improved morbidity and mortality rates for the hospital and their medical staff.

You may contact him at *RGold@DCBAInc.com.*

Documentation Strategies to Support Severity of Illness: Ensure an Accurate Professional Profile, Second Edition

Introduction

Doctors in the United States are becoming more aware of the value of clinical data and the relationships between their professional profiles and the ICD-9-CM and CPT codes they assign, or those assigned for them by others. Certainly, internists are aware of the value of personal professional billing codes, and surgeons are aware of their morbidity and mortality rates. These entities all revolve around the ICD-9-CM codes assigned for diagnoses, treatments, and procedures performed. If the clinical documentation and, thus, the codes do not accurately and specifically represent the work you do, someone can be inconvenienced—if not actually hurt—with data that poorly reflect on the practitioner's quality of care.

Professional organizations have started to work to help their physician members understand how clinical documentation and the ICD-9-CM codes derived from that documentation affect quality of care, in addition to the other effects previously mentioned. Physicians must under-

complexity of the physician's medical decision-making reflects the complexity of the patient, and the terms that physicians use in the medical record—whether in the hospital, their offices, or in the nursing home—lead to code assignments that either do or do not inform the database that they know their patients.

All physicians took courses in pathology and physiology and learned about causes of symptoms and specific etiologies of disease manifestations. However, physicians often take shortcuts when they document in their patients' medical records, and those shortcuts hurt the United States and its overall healthcare system.

The Uniform Hospital Discharge Data Set (UHDDS) requires hospitals to report conditions that affect patient care and require clinical evaluation, therapeutic treatment, diagnostic procedures, extended length of hospital stay, and increased nursing care/monitoring. Identifying these components of the conditions adds to the complexity of your medical decision-making and enhances your severity profiles.

Physicians and the hospital health information management (HIM) or medical record department must communicate with each other. The HIM coding staff must have the opportunity to ask physicians questions or to request clarification when clinical documentation is not specific.

This handbook will help you understand many of the specific diagnosis-related issues—and relieve the physician of much of the rework associated with utilization review, case management, HIM/medical records issues, and questions from those who oversee your work.

Note that this handbook is not all-inclusive, but serves as a guide to improving clinical documentation and to capturing severity, acuity, and risk of mortality for the patients you serve.

Acute Myocardial Infarction

Classification of acute myocardial infarction (MI) has two major categories:

- **Type 1:** Acute coronary occlusion by thrombus, embolism, or ruptured atherosclerotic plaque

- **Type 2:** Demand acute MI

Additionally, true MIs are classified as follows:

- **Type 3:** Associated with sudden cardiac death, such that the physician does not know whether an MI caused a fatal arrhythmia or an arrhythmia caused the MI.

- **Type 4:** MIs that occur related to a current angioplasty with or without stent. Depending on the clinical circumstances, it may not require intervention if it is small or it may be significant and require further intervention.

- **Type 5:** MIs that occur related to a current coronary artery bypass procedure.

In Types 4 and 5, if not clinically significant, no complication code should be considered. If increased treatment or other intervention for an adverse patient outcome from the post-procedural MI is required, then a cardiac complication of surgery code should be assigned to track it.

Result

- Non-ST-elevation MI (**NSTEMI**), which can occur because of Type 1 or Type 2 mechanism

- ST-elevation MI (**STEMI**), which usually occurs with Type 1 mechanism but can also occur with Type 4 or 5 events

Clinical criteria

- Symptoms of acute MI (either typical presentation with chest pain or atypical without chest pain) and

- There is a significant spike in troponin level with at least one reading higher than top normal for the laboratory. Three equally elevated troponins do not signify an acute MI—this usually identifies a chronic condition.

Documentation needs
Acute episode

- Did the patient, after workup, likely have an MI (NSTEMI or STEMI)? (Documentation may state acute coronary syndrome with troponinemia or demand ischemia.)

- If STEMI, was there cardiogenic shock or new left bundle branch block? (Check whether vital signs show significantly low blood pressure and whether a ventricular assist device or pressors were used.)

- If demand MI, what was the causative factor? (Atrial fibrillation [AF] with rapid ventricular response [RVR] or other tachyarrhythmia, severe chronic anemia or acute anemia, and the cause of the anemia or hypoxia, and from what source, etc.)

- Did the patient present with congestive heart failure (CHF)? Seek clarification if acute. (Check whether the brain natriuretic peptide [BNP] is elevated, if there is presence of rales or shortness of breath, or if there is x-ray showing pulmonary edema.)

- Did the patient develop pericarditis or other post-MI symptoms such as post-MI fever or post-MI leukocytosis (signs of Dressler's syndrome), or was there post-MI angina? (Document whether there is continued chest pain after the MI and its cause.)

- Did the patient have an arrhythmia during the hospital stay that was not documented and that may or may not have required treatment? If so, name that arrhythmia and the decision-making.

- When documentation is not clear as to the acuity of the MI:
  - Is this the first hospitalization for that acute MI?

- Did the patient have the MI prior to admission, or did this event occur after admission? Document the principal diagnoses that actually led to the decision to admit.

- Was there a second MI during this or a recent hospitalization and did it occur within 4 weeks of a previous one?

Background heart disease (see Heart Failure)

- Does the patient have background heart disease with right heart failure (chronic cor pulmonale) or chronic left ventricular systolic or diastolic heart failure (check echo for ejection fraction [EF] and modeling of hypertrophy [diastolic dysfunction with normal EF] or dilation of left ventricle [systolic dysfunction with EF + 40%])?

- Is it due to ischemic cardiomyopathy, valvular disease, hypertensive heart disease, alcoholic cardiomyopathy, amyloid heart, viral cardiomyopathy, toxic cardiomyopathy (and from what drug), hypertrophic cardiomyopathy, or unknown cause?

- Document your answer(s) to the question(s) in progress notes and upon discharge.

Adverse Effects of Medications

Background and clinical implications

Sometimes, medications have side effects on organs that can lead to discomfort or functional abnormalities that will mimic other diseases, such as nausea and vomiting, diarrhea, or drop in blood pressure with syncope or acute renal failure. Sometimes, there are cumulative effects of drugs where one will not cause a significant abnormality but, along with other drugs, can lead to confusion that another disease might exist, such as with alteration of consciousness or shortness of breath. And sometimes, a patient will have a life-threatening event as an undesired effect that rarely occurs in the general population.

Finally, in the face of the desired effect of a drug, another condition that a patient has gets significantly worse, such as gastrointestinal bleeding, hematuria in a patient on warfarin, or acute respiratory failure from worsening chronic obstructive pulmonary disease (COPD) in a hypertensive patient on beta blockers.

- When a drug is given to the proper patient in the proper dosage and taken properly, a clinical problem that occurs is called an adverse effect. If the wrong patient takes the medication or the right patient takes an overdose, that is considered a poisoning for the purpose of capturing coded data.

- When the medical workup demonstrates that the patient's presenting symptoms are due to side effects or adverse effects of a medicine taken properly, the presenting disease is sequenced as the principal diagnosis and an E-code (adverse effect code) is assigned later to show what drug or class of drug led to the effect.

Note: **Warfarin** (Coumadin™) **toxicity** is not poisoning unless the patient took the wrong dosage. The effect (high prothrombin time or international normalized ratio [INR] level) or whatever is bleeding is the diagnosis along with a V code for long-term use of anticoagulants.

Phenytoin (Dilantin™) **toxicity** is not poisoning unless the patient took the wrong dosage. The symptoms the patient presented with will be the principal diagnosis (e.g., nausea and vomiting, alteration of consciousness).

The most important detail is the **documented link of the presenting symptoms** or **the worsening of the presentation to the specific drug(s)**.

Documentation needs

- Document the patient's signs and symptoms of the adverse effect of the medication you believe is the cause, and use the term "due to."

- Document drug-drug interactions; specifically, name the drugs and the adverse effect.

- Document patients who take multiple drugs and who may be influenced by multiple side effects. Specify whether this is the cause of specific symptoms.

- Document predisposing factors, such as other diseases the patient has, dietary issues, or over-the-counter drug use.

- When respiratory depression is due to drug use, specify/document whether the case involved proper dosage, overdosage, or use of illicit or illegal drugs. (These are poisonings rather than adverse effects because there is usually no prescribed dosage by a physician.)

Alcohol/Substance Use/Abuse

Background

Patients may present to the hospital with symptoms related to current use of alcohol or illicit drugs, or with other conditions that can be tied to the patient's recent acute or habitual use of these substances. The specificity of the pattern of use and the link of the symptoms to the substance use is fundamental.

- **Abuse** implies overuse of alcohol or any use of illicit drugs without implication of dependence. Abuse can be *episodic* (e.g., only on weekends) or *continuous* (e.g., daily). These are classified by the specific drug or drug group used by the patient (e.g., marijuana, hallucinogens, opioids, cocaine).

- **Dependence** is similarly divided by overuse of alcohol or other illicit substances, but implies that it is more than "recreational" and the patient's lifestyle is impacted by the presence or absence of the dependent substance. Again, this is divided in the coding classification by *continuous* or *episodic* use.

Documentation needs

- Clarify/document in the record whether a patient sometimes drinks alcohol but does not have an abuse or dependence problem (e.g., cite "social drinking" and volume of wine, beer, or other).

- Specify/document whether the patient has a history of alcohol problems, whether this is a case of periodic or episodic abuse (e.g., weekend drinker), or whether the patient is alcohol dependent.

- Specify/document whether the patient has other body system effects of alcohol or drug abuse or dependence and name the related disease process.

- Document whether you believe the patient is an occasional abuser or is dependent on alcohol or illegal or controlled drugs.

- Document whether the patient suffers from substance abuse and name the substance. Writing (+) coc or (+) barb or (-) ETOH means nothing clinically. Coding staff may not apply codes from a positive lab test per guidelines.

- Identify whether there is a link between the identified drug abuse or dependence and organ malfunction, such as alcoholic cardiomyopathy, alcoholic cirrhosis, or chest pain due to cocaine abuse.

Anemia

Clinical criteria

Clinical criteria include a hemoglobin level that is below low normal for your laboratory—use 10 as a general rule. A drop in hemoglobin level without achieving anemia does not require questioning here, but may require defining the cause of the drop in hemoglobin.

Mechanisms

- **Congenital disease**—sickle cell, thalassemia, spherocytosis, ellipticytosis, glucose-6-phosphatase dehydrogenase deficiency

- **Nutrient deficiency**—iron deficiency (microcytic, hypochromic red cells), vitamin B_{12} (macrocytic anemia), severe protein malnutrition

- **Chronic blood loss**—gastrointestinal (GI) blood loss, chronic hematuria, menometrorrhagia

- **Acute blood loss**—due to a disease, such as acute GI bleed, rupture of aneurysm or other vessel tear, spleen or liver rupture, severe scalp laceration, fracture of femur, or associated with an operation involving large volumes of blood loss such as aortic aneurysm surgery, liver surgery

- **Complication of a surgical procedure**—operation usually associated with small volumes of blood loss may entail massive blood loss due to inadvertent events (e.g., tear of a major vein, avulsion of spleen, unplanned entry into the aorta or major artery), which may result in anemia from acute blood loss

- **Chronic kidney disease (CKD)**—usually stage 3 or higher with glomerular filtration rate (GFR) + 45 mL/min

- **Specific other chronic disease**—such as hepatitis, chronic osteomyelitis; name condition

- **Chemotherapy**—check whether platelets and white count also low in cases of transient pancytopenia or long-term aplastic anemia; name chemotherapy drug

- **Bone marrow malignancy**—neoplasm in the bone marrow or of the bone marrow

- Myelodysplastic condition

- Hemodilution only

Thought processes

- Patient may have multiple factors at play at any time—you will need to specify/document these

- A significant drop in hemoglobin may be indicative of acute blood loss but the patient may not develop anemia

- It could start within the normal range for the patient's gender and drop to below normal (below 10), in which case it is reasonable to determine that the patient has anemia due to acute blood loss

- It could start below normal and drop significantly lower, in which case it may be anemia due to some chronic cause, in addition to anemia due to acute blood loss

Acute GI bleed, acute menorrhagia, acute onset of gross hematuria, or **acute retroperitoneal hematoma** all imply "blood loss;" therefore, no additional clarification is needed to determine that there was blood loss, but you do need to include the "acute" or document that it just happened.

A low hemoglobin level with no significant change implies a chronic anemic condition. Only cases associated with known bleeding are eligible to be called anemia due to chronic blood loss.

Note: Newly found "iron deficiency anemia" in an elderly patient is cancer of the right colon until proven otherwise.

Documentation needs

- Document whether the patient has anemia due to blood loss from a disease process, and name that disease process (e.g., anemia due to acute blood loss from fracture of the femur; anemia due to chronic blood loss from a right colon cancer).

- Document whether the patient is anemic from another cause, such as end-stage renal disease (ESRD) or bone marrow suppression, and document an explanation of the link, such as anemia of ESRD, anemia from chemotherapy, anemia of bone marrow suppression in myeloma, etc.

- In addition to anemia, clarify in your documentation whether a patient has transient pancytopenia due to chemotherapeutic agents or other specific drug, or whether it has resulted in long-term or permanent aplastic anemia.

- Document whether a patient develops anemia from excessive blood loss from the GI tract or the urinary tract, due to retroperitoneal bleed, during surgery due to a true hematologic problem, or due to being on long-term anticoagulants.

- Document the factors of which you are aware that have contributed to the patient's case of "multifactorial" anemia and identify each one.

- Document whether a patient has excessive blood loss during a procedure due to a complication that occurred, such as inadvertent entry into the femoral vein during a herniorrhaphy.

Chest Pain/Angina

Chest pain can have numerous causes. The most important thing for a physician to determine is if the chest pain represents an acute MI. Once that is ruled out (usually by electrocardiogram or rise in troponin level), other cardiac or noncardiac causes of chest pain must be determined. Often, the specific cause is never identified.

Cardiac causes

- Acute MI (see Acute Myocardial Infarction)

- **Unstable angina** due to CAD or due to:

    – Aortic stenosis

    – Hypertrophic cardiomyopathy

- Pulmonary artery hypertension

- Severe anemia (acute or progressive chronic—pain relieved with transfusion)

- Tachyarrhythmia (AF with RVR, supraventricular tachycardia, etc.—pain relieved with slowing heart rate)

- Hypertensive emergency (accelerated or malignant hypertension—pain relieved with dropping blood pressure)

- Thyroid storm

- Any shock or significant hypovolemia

- Stable angina

- Pericarditis (with or without effusion)

- Myocarditis

Noncardiac causes

- Pulmonary embolism (from deep vein thrombosis, fat embolism, air embolism)

- Costochondritis (reproducible pain with pressure on costal cartilage)

- Gastroesophageal reflux

- Rib fracture or other chest trauma

- Pneumonia/pleurisy

- Lung cancer

- Acute cholecystitis or hepatitis

Documentation needs

- Document the origin of the chest pain (i.e., cardiac, noncardiac).

- If angina, specify/document whether it is stable, unstable, acute MI, acute pericarditis, myocardial contusion, etc.

- Document the primary source of the angina, if known (e.g., CAD, aortic stenosis, hypertrophic cardiomyopathy, pulmonary artery hypertension, Prinzmetal coronary spasm).

- Document whether the pain represents secondary cause of unstable angina and specify whether it is due to tachyarrhythmia, bradycardia, anemia, or metabolic demands, such as thyrotoxicosis, etc.

- Specify/document whether the chest pain is related to a condition, such as musculoskeletal, pleuritic, gastroesophageal reflux disease (GERD), gallbladder, Tietze syndrome, etc., if known.

Chronic Obstructive Pulmonary Disease

COPD can be a chronic stable condition or present with acute symptoms of shortness of breath, cough, and frequently, wheezing (called exacerbation of COPD).

Causes

- Inhalation of smoke or chemicals (cigarettes, anthracosis, other irritants)

- Repeated aspiration of gastric content

- Prolonged, repeated severe asthma attacks

- Emphysema

- Bronchiectasis

- Severity of chronic COPD ranges from mild to severe. If a patient has severe COPD or end-stage COPD, presence of chronic respiratory failure must be considered.

- Severity of acute exacerbation ranges from outpatient treatment to treatments in the emergency department to acute respiratory failure, which may require ventilatory support.

Clinical criteria

- Acute respiratory failure

- Documented evidence of difficulty in breathing: use of accessory muscles of respiration, inability to speak more than two-word sentences, tachypnea (over 24 breaths/minute), cyanosis

- Hypoxemic (Type 1) respiratory failure: SaO_2 cannot be maintained at 90% with 6 L of oxygen or $pO_2 < 60$ on room air

- Hypercapnic (Type 2) respiratory failure: $pH < 7.30$, $pCO_2 > 50$

- Chronic respiratory failure

  - pH normal with $pCO_2 > 50$

  - Polycythemia

  - Chronic cor pulmonale

  - Clubbing of fingers

Documentation needs

- Document whether the patient has acute bronchitis, acute exacerbation of chronic bronchitis, stable COPD, or other chronic lung disease.

- Document whether the patient has acute exacerbation of chronic asthmatic bronchitis when chronic asthma has led to chronic lung disease.

- Document whether the patient had acute respiratory failure upon admission, even if it did not require intubation.

- Document whether the patient has chronic respiratory failure and needs home oxygen and other treatments while meeting above criteria.

- Document the likely etiology of this acute event (e.g., allergy, cold, viral or bacterial bronchitis, pneumonia).

- Document whether this patient's exacerbation was likely caused by aspiration (microaspiration related to GERD or laryngeal dysfunction, etc.) and requires evaluation or treatment of the aspiration risk (aspiration bronchitis or aspiration pneumonitis).

Comfort Measures Only

Rationale

A patient's and family's desires regarding the extent of intervention for a terminal or dying patient while in the hospital has many levels. The assignment of **do not resuscitate (DNR)** status may vary from providing all care as needed for all conditions that the patient develops short of intubation and mechanical ventilation to refusal of any medical interaction whatsoever. The assignment of **Comfort Measures Only** is a status usually arrived at with coordination of stated desires of the patient, the family, the physician, and pastoral support.

Palliative services may be provided by a hospital team for any patient who requires ongoing treatment after discharge. The mere involvement of the palliative care team does *not* qualify for Comfort Measures Only. Palliative care that is provided to prepare the patient for imminent death *does* qualify.

Comfort measures may include hydration, pain control, drugs to control seizure activity, or any intervention to prevent the dying patient from becoming agitated and more uncomfortable. Antibiotics and any other drug used to treat a condition other than to keep the patient comfortable will be discontinued. Often, the situation will involve removing the patient from a ventilator and allowing death to ensue.

Documentation needs

- Document medical staff communication with the family (whether by the consulting physician, chaplain, palliative care, etc.) regarding "withdrawal of life support" or "keep the patient comfortable" or "agreed to let the patient die with dignity." Additionally, there should be existing documentation regarding DNR (or other similar terminology) within the medical record. Clarify whether this documentation meets your definition of Comfort Measures Only or indicates intervention to be provided to the patient in case of change in status.

- If you request a palliative care consult (or inpatient hospice consult), document discussion with the patient or family and others regarding discontinuation of care. If you intend to maintain patient comfort with no further intervention, clarify whether the intent is Comfort Measures Only or some limitation of response to change as in a DNR or other status.

Comorbidities (Comorbid Conditions)

Rationale

Severity-adjusted data is being collected on physicians as much as on hospitals. Severity-adjusted mortality risk or complication risk for surgeries will impact the surgical specialties more than ever before. When the physician in charge of the patient's care can document all of the patient's diseases on admission to the hospital, all the coexisting conditions, whether the conditions are acute or chronic but are being treated, the severity of illness, risk of mortality, and complexity of medical decision-making are properly reflected.

For medical specialties, the comorbidities (patient's present diseases that are being managed, even though stable) affect the level of facility or professional billing for all admissions.

For surgical specialties, the comorbidities (other diseases that could potentially impact wound healing, recovery from anesthesia, and resistance to infection) are important data for the National Surgical Quality Improvement Project and for the Society for Thoracic Surgery database.

Physicians should name all diseases for which they are ordering medications, even home medications, because they are responsible for the treatment of those diseases while the patient is in the hospital, regardless of the service for which the patient is admitted.

Documentation needs

- Document in the history and physical (H&P) whether the patient has other diseases that you or another physician are following, and name those diseases.

- Document in the H&P the medications that the patient is currently taking and for what diseases they are prescribed.

- Document all conditions (risk factors) that exist that could affect the patient's ability to tolerate surgery, result in problems during or after an operation, or affect the hospitalization.

- Name/document a diagnosis whenever the patient's condition changes while he or she is in the hospital and you order tests or treatments.

- Document in the operative note any complications that occur during the operation and require corrective action.

Complications (Postoperative)

Background

Clinical conditions may be noted in the time period after an intervention, whether major surgical or procedural, that may not have been identified prior to the procedure. Sometimes, it is a matter of getting a more complete history of present illnesses after a surgical procedure has been performed. Sometimes, it will be a manifestation of the disease for which the surgery was performed. Other times, it will be an event that occurred in the operating suite due to the anesthesia or surgery.

Complications of surgery are conditions that follow an intervention and were caused by that intervention. Therefore, it becomes important to determine whether the diagnostic term reported in the postoperative period actually represented one of the above circumstances rather than having been a complication of the surgery. The coding data captures complications through the ICD-9-CM codes, which come from the clinical documentation.

Surgeons are measured by their complication statistics (i.e., morbidity and mortality rates). If they do cause harm, it is important to capture the cause and the effect. Often, people learn from mistakes or adverse events.

Anemia that may be found after surgery for a fracture of the neck of the femur is often due to the fracture, not the surgery. It could be referred to as **anemia due to acute blood loss from the femur fracture**. Similarly, anemia following surgery for a GI bleed may be referred to as **anemia due to acute blood loss from the bleeding diverticulum**.

After **perforation of intestine** (diverticulum, appendix, gallbladder), ileus will occur because of the perforation and will prolong the postoperative recovery, but it represents ileus due to the perforated bowel. Adynamic or paralytic ileus is a normal consequence of an abdominal surgery and usually resolves in three to four days. Ileus that prolongs the stay considerably beyond that or which results in reinsertion of a nasogastric tube may, indeed, be a complication of the surgery. However, be sure to confirm that the patient did not have intestinal motility issues prior to the operative procedure, such as diabetic gastroparesis, which may have been the true cause of the prolonged ileus.

Events such as **wound infection, wound breakdown, excessive hemorrhage** from the wound and **hematomas** of significant size to require active treatment or significantly prolonged observation, **seromas, abscesses** after clean-clean surgery, and **pneumonia** (not present on admission or developing on admission) are always surgical complications.

If a surgeon or an internist who is following the case uses the term "postoperative" preceding a diagnosis (e.g., postoperative urinary retention, postoperative atelectasis), the code assignment may well turn out to be a complication code. It becomes important to ensure the coder (as well as the surgeon) that several analytic processes must be followed prior to assigning a complication code to the case:

- The diagnostic condition was not caused by patient disease or medications

- The diagnostic condition met UHDDS criteria as a valid secondary diagnosis (clinically insignificant events should not be assigned complication codes)

- The diagnostic condition was unavoidable due to complexity of the operative procedure, as with massive lysis of complex adhesions and inadvertent laceration of the serosa or entry into the bowel

- The diagnostic condition was not a complication of the anesthesia

- The diagnostic condition was not present on admission

- The diagnostic condition did not precede the procedure

- The diagnostic condition was not a normal part of events that occur following a procedure, and virtually all patients undergoing this procedure do not acquire that condition

- Documentation of "postoperative" _____ was found in the progress notes. Please clarify whether this was a complication of the procedure or provide some etiology to explain its presence (e.g., caused by the disease, caused by anesthesia, was present on admission but not identified at that time).

Coronary Artery Disease

It is important to identify atherosclerosis of the coronary arteries as the cause either of a presenting symptom or of the disease process being treated. Specificity of the particular vessel involved, when known, is also crucial for data analysis. Coronary artery disease (CAD) is divided into the following:

- Native vessel (always the right designation when the patient has had no coronary artery surgery)

- Vein bypass

- Synthetic bypass

- Artery bypass (internal mammary)

- Native vessel of transplant heart

- Bypass vessel of transplant heart

- Unknown, native, or bypass vessel

Sometimes, long-term atherosclerotic disease of the coronaries can lead to long-term functional abnormality of the entire heart and result in heart failure (ischemic cardiomyopathy).

When there has been a stent inserted in a coronary artery, it is important to designate whether obstruction at the stent is likely due to progression of the atherosclerosis in the stent or there was premature blockage due to malpositioning of the stent (in-stent stenosis or end-stent stenosis).

Documentation needs

- Specify/document whether the obstructive disease found in the coronaries is the cause of the patient's chest pain or suspected to be the cause.

- Specify/document whether the cause of the patient's documented cardiomyopathy is coronary occlusive disease (ischemic cardiomyopathy) or some other known cause (e.g., hypertension, valvular disease, viral cardiomyopathy, amyloid).

- Specify/document in the medical record of your patient with documented coronary artery bypass grafting (CABG) whether the symptoms are due to disease of the remaining native vessels or due to occlusion of bypass vein or artery or other graft. Name the vessel or graft material if known.

- Specify/document whether your patient has had angioplasty and a stent, and whether the current symptoms are due to occlusion of other native vessels or of the stent.

- Specify/document the cause if a patient with CAD developed unstable angina because of anemia or tachyarrhythmia or other secondary cause.

Debridement

Several treatment modalities are available for debridement. Debridement may be part of cleaning of an open wound in preparation for closure, of a comminuted fracture, or of a burn in preparation for applying a skin graft. None of these requires specific documentation.

Within ICD-9-CM, **excisional debridement** is the excision of devitalized tissue, necrosis, and/or slough using sharp instruments, such as scalpel, scissors, laser, or curette, down to healthy tissue to enable speedier healing. It is imperative for the provider to document the deepest tissue actually removed (skin and subcutaneous tissue, tendon sheath, muscle, and/or bone).

ICD-9-CM classifies that **nonexcisional debridement** can be exemplified with use of forceps, water jet, chemicals, or wet-to-dry dressings.

The diagnosis of the lesion(s) actually debrided is essential for proper classification (e.g., burn, infected surgical wound, pressure ulcer, arterial ulcer, venous stasis ulcer, diabetic neuropathic or vascular ulcer).

Documentation needs

- Whether in the operating room or at the bedside, document whenever the procedure was done sharply (with scissors or knife) with a goal of excising necrotic tissue from a wound, infection, or burn down to healthy granulation tissue.

- Document whether the procedure was merely cleaning up the edges of a laceration prior to closure.

- Document whether the procedure represented removing abraded, dirty tissue, or bone fragments prior to closure or fixation of an open fracture.

- Clarify/document in the medical record whether the procedure was debridement of toenails to differentiate it from debridement of a foot ulcer, for example.

- Designate/document when a method other than sharp technique was used.

- Clarify/document the deepest tissue actually removed and the size of the area of the lesion debrided.

Dementia/Delirium/Encephalopathy

Background

Alteration of mental status (time, place, and person) or **alteration of consciousness** (awake, unresponsive, comatose) can have multiple possible causes, some of which can be life-threatening and require immediate evaluation and initiation of treatment and some with which the patients will live the rest of their lives. From poisonings or overdoses of narcotic, sedative, tranquilizer, or illicit drugs to septic metabolic encephalopathy to senile dementia, the workup and diagnosis after workup becomes very important.

Definitions

Dementia is a long-term condition and is due to progressive destruction of brain cells. Dementia is a loss of brain function that occurs with certain diseases. It affects memory, thinking, language, judgment, and behavior. Most types of dementia are nonreversible (degenerative).

Alzheimer's disease is the most common type of dementia. Lewy body disease is a leading cause of dementia in elderly adults. People with this condition have abnormal protein structures in certain areas of the brain. Dementia also can be due to many small strokes. This is called vascular dementia. The following medical conditions also can lead to dementia:

- Parkinson's disease

- Multiple sclerosis

- Huntington's disease

- Pick's disease

- Progressive supranuclear palsy

Delirium is a condition of acute onset and short duration that may be a manifestation of many conditions. When it is such a manifestation, it is a symptom and, as such, one should determine the cause. It may be a symptom of a transient encephalopathy, such as hypernatremic encephalopathy; it may be a symptom of change in location of a patient with Alzheimer's dementia who becomes delirious when no longer in a familiar surrounding; or it may be due to the effect of alcohol or anti-Parkinson drugs or steroids or other medications. It needs specificity and should *not* be sought as a diagnosis. It is a manifestation of something else.

Encephalopathy is a term for any diffuse disease of the brain that alters brain function or structure. Encephalopathy may be caused by an infectious agent (bacteria, virus, or prion), metabolic or mitochondrial dysfunction, brain tumor or increased pressure in the skull, prolonged exposure to toxic elements (including solvents, drugs, radiation, paints, industrial chemicals, and certain metals), chronic progressive trauma, poor nutrition, or lack of oxygen or blood flow to the brain. Common neurological symptoms are progressive loss of memory and cognitive ability, subtle personality changes, inability to concentrate, lethargy, and progressive loss of consciousness. Other neurological symptoms may include myoclonus (involuntary twitching of a muscle or group of muscles), nystagmus (rapid, involuntary eye movement), tremor, muscle atrophy and weakness, dementia, seizures, and loss of ability to swallow or speak.

Encephalopathy is divided into three major groups:

1. Hypoxic encephalopathy

- Circulatory arrest

- Disorders associated with cardiac procedures (e.g., percutaneous transluminal coronary angioplasty, CABG, valve replacement)—rule out stroke

2. **Metabolic encephalopathy**

- Associated with sepsis

- Hepatic, uremic, hyper- or hyponatremic encephalopathies, etc.

3. **Toxic encephalopathy**

- Iatrogenic disorders (chemotherapy, steroid-induced, vaccine-induced, complication of transplant)

- Lead exposure, toxic solvents

Other named encephalopathies:

- Mitochondrial encephalopathy

- Glycine encephalopathy

- Hashimoto's encephalopathy

- Transmissible spongiform encephalopathy

- Neonatal hypoxemic ischemic encephalopathy

What is *not* encephalopathy:

- Intentional sedation from medication

- Being drunk or high on improper use of drugs

- Vasovagal syncope

- Transient cerebrovascular hypoperfusion

- Stroke or transient ischemic attack (TIA)

- Progressive dementia (name cause)

- Transient delirium in an elderly patient with chronic, degenerative brain disease due to unfamiliarity with surroundings while in the hospital

Be aware of stroke causing change in awareness, subdural bleed, head trauma, TIA, syncope due to transient hypoperfusion of the brain (as in bradycardia, vasovagal syncope), generalized hypoxemia (as in pulmonary embolism), or other specific causes and link the presentation to the cause.

Documentation needs

- Clarify/document whether the patient's altered mental status was due to one of the conditions named in the record (name which one) or supply the cause, if known.

- Document the likely cause of a patient's delirium, which is often a symptom of something else, such as generalized cerebrovascular ischemia, Alzheimer's disease, or toxic effects of drugs, etc. When you can identify the likely cause of the patient's presentation and elect to address treatment or care to that cause, document that relationship in the medical record.

- Document whether the patient likely has an organic cause or psychological cause of the presentation of altered mental status. An elderly patient may have psychological problems that supersede the decreased brain function from dementia as well. Be sure to clarify this information.

- Document whether you think there is infection, sepsis, dehydration, or specific organ failure that is causing the delirium and whether it represents that specific encephalopathy. Be specific when clarifying the relationship between that process and the mental status change.

- Document the relationship of the mental status change to any other disease process.

Femur Fracture—Treatment

Background

- The trauma leading to fracture of a femur can vary depending on the patient's bone health. Patients with bone diseases may suffer femoral fractures with minimal trauma. **Osteoporosis** is the No. 1 cause of such fractures in the United States. When a bone is fractured with inadequate trauma to have fractured a normal bone and the condition is known, the result is a **pathologic fracture.**

- Repair of a fractured femur depends on the viability of the bony fragments and the location along the femur. Some fractures require no surgery because they are well aligned and the patient is not likely to walk because of concomitant disease or the patient is too sick to undergo surgery. Some patients with risk of aseptic necrosis of the head of the femur who are immobile already may undergo removal of the head and neck of the femur with no reconstruction (Girdlestone procedure).

- Fractures around the neck of the femur are classified as **pertrochanteric, intertrochanteric,** or **subtrochanteric.** Orthopedists will select a CPT code for open treatment of such fractures depending on which portion of the neck of the femur was fractured. They are all open surgery codes. ICD-9-CM classifies open surgery on the basis of if and when a reduction was performed. An alternative surgical approach is to perform a total replacement of the femoral head if it is assumed that the arterial supply to the head of the femur will lead to aseptic necrosis.

- **Fractures of the shaft** of the femur or **supracondylar fractures** are often treated with insertion of an intramedullary rod. Again, it is imperative to determine whether fracture reduction was performed and whether it was done before or after the skin incision.

- **Femoral fractures,** regardless of whether the patient goes to the operating room, are occasionally associated with other conditions, such as anemia due to acute blood loss from the fracture site itself—which may or may not lead to anemia and may or may not require blood transfusion—and the occurrence of fatty pulmonary emboli from the fracture site or venous pulmonary emboli from the immobility.

Documentation needs

- Document in the operative/procedure note whether you reduced the fracture at all (impacted and in good alignment) and whether reduction was achieved prior to or after the incision.

- Document whether the patient lost enough blood from the fracture to drop the hematocrit to a level consistent with anemia that would warrant follow-up, monitoring, or transfusion. This is not a complication of surgery—it is anemia due to acute blood loss from the fracture.

- Document other chronic, stable conditions that are under treatment, even if they are followed by another physician while the patient is in the hospital.

- Document a diagnosis for any treatments instituted in the postoperative phase, such as acute urinary retention, atelectasis, or volume overload—don't simply treat the condition without naming it. If the condition is due to an identifiable disease, make the link (e.g., acute urinary retention due to benign prostatic hyperplasia, atelectasis due to morbid obesity). Do not call it "postoperative urinary retention" or "postoperative atelectasis."

Gastrointestinal Bleed

GI bleeds can be slow, chronic conditions or acute, hemorrhagic events. In the acute GI bleed, it may be of:

- Low enough volume or rate of bleed to not cause hemodynamic instability—no specific documentation is needed

- Enough volume change to lead to tachycardia and hypotension, but not enough to cause significant organ hypoperfusion—reflects hypovolemia

- Large volume with sufficient hypotension to cause organ damage—reflective of hemorrhagic shock

Initial identification of the potential site of the bleed can be surmised by the character of the bleed:

- Bright red blood through the anus is most frequently lower GI bleed

- Bright red blood in vomitus is most frequently rapid upper GI bleed

- Coffee-ground vomitus often signifies slower upper GI bleed

- Black blood in stool (melena) signifies that the blood originated above the duodenum (esophagus or stomach)

Be aware that bleeding gums, nosebleed, or another source not associated with the GI tract, as well as ingestion of bismuth subsalicylate or drinking blood can cause heme-positive stool.

Link findings on endoscopy to the bleed, if possible. Sometimes, pathologic findings are visualized but may not be actively bleeding at the time of the procedure, yet the endoscopist might consider them the likely source of the bleed. If you cannot locate the source, it is more appropriate to identify whether it is thought to be an upper GI bleed or a lower GI bleed rather than just documenting "melena," "hematochezia," or "vomiting blood."

Be sure to evaluate the patient's hemoglobin and hematocrit upon admission and throughout the hospital stay. Identify whether anemia ever develops. It is important to determine whether the patient was anemic on admission and stayed anemic (until transfused, if transfusion is necessary). That anemia may be due to chronic blood loss or some other source of anemia (see Anemia). If there is significant drop in hemoglobin and hematocrit, it is likely an acute bleed. A patient may have chronic anemia due to kidney disease (or some other cause) and acute anemia (progressive drop in red blood count) due to acute GI blood loss.

Documentation needs

- Document whether you think that the patient's GI bleed is causing anemia. Document whether it is anemia due to acute blood loss or due to chronic blood loss.

- Document whether you suspect that the cause is upper GI or lower GI until you have done studies to prove it. Remember, "rectal bleeds" originate in the rectum. If the bleed is melena or hematochezia, use those terms instead until you determine the source.

- Clarify/document in the record whether tests indicate a GI tract lesion and whether you think the lesion is the origin of a GI bleed.

- Specify/document in the record which lesion you believe to be the cause of the bleed if you discover two or more lesions on your workup.

- Specify/document that you don't know the cause of the GI bleed if your workup reveals several possible lesions or no lesions and you still do not know the possible etiology of the GI blood loss.

Heart Failure

Heart failure can be an acute condition requiring acute medical attention or a chronic, background condition. Heart failure can involve the left side of the heart only, the right side of the heart only, or both sides. The traditionally known concept of **CHF** is caused by left heart failure, with backup of fluid into the lungs. With right heart failure, there is backup into the legs with edema, the abdomen with ascites, the liver with chronic passive congestion or cardiac cirrhosis, and the veins overall with jugular venous distension.

Cardiomyopathy

Chronic heart failure can have many causes, including ischemic cardiomyopathy, valvular heart disease, hypertensive heart disease, alcoholic cardiomyopathy, hypertrophic cardiomyopathy (with or without outflow obstruction), and amyloidosis of the heart. Just because a patient has a cardiomyopathy does not mean that there is heart failure.

Dysfunction

When the left ventricle does not work properly, there is dysfunction. Chronic dysfunction comes from modeling of the left ventricular wall either with stiffness and inability to fill adequately during diastole (diastolic dysfunction) or with dilatation causing weak contractions during systole (systolic dysfunction). Just because there is dysfunction does not mean that there is heart failure.

Left heart failure

When a patient with a cardiomyopathy (any of the previously mentioned processes) and dysfunction of the left ventricle first develops symptoms of heart failure, the patient has a chronic heart failure from then on.

Right heart failure

Dilation or hypertrophy of the right ventricle can occur because of all the same cardiomyopathies as in left heart failure, except for different valves (tricuspid and pulmonic) and a different source of hypertension (pulmonary hypertension, either primary or secondary to some other disease).

Acute left heart failure

Usually, this is acute diastolic dysfunction with fluid overloading the lungs. This can occur as an exacerbation of a patient's chronic heart failure status or be an independent event with no background left heart failure. Conditions such as tachyarrhythmia (AF with RVR or supraventricular or ventricular tachycardia), an acute ischemic event (coronary occlusive MI or demand MI), or an accelerated hypertension or Takotsubo syndrome can cause acute left heart failure regardless of whether the patient has background chronic heart failure. Most hospital admissions are for acute exacerbation (or decompensation) of chronic heart failure. Documentation of the chronic state drives the proper coding. Examples are exacerbation of chronic diastolic heart failure with LVH and normal EF, or decompensation of chronic systolic failure with dilated LV and EF + 40%.

Left ventricular echo or ventriculogram

When the left ventricle is thickened (left ventricular hypertrophy) or stiff and has a normal ejection fraction (over 40%, usually 55%–70%) in the presence of documented heart failure, it probably signifies **chronic left ventricular diastolic failure.** When the left ventricle is dilated and has an EF + 40% with documented CHF, the condition is likely **chronic left ventricular systolic failure.**

Need to know:

- Left ventricular failure or right ventricular failure, or both?

- If left ventricular failure, is it acute CHF (and the mechanism causing it), chronic heart failure (and the causative cardiomyopathy), or decompensation of a chronic heart failure?

Classification of heart failure

- **New York Heart Association Classes 1–4:** Class 1 is preheart failure; Classes 2 and 3 justify insertion of a defibrillator when associated with systolic dysfunction; Class 4 is terminal end-stage heart failure.

- **American Heart Association Stages 1–4:** Stage 1 is cardiomyopathy—there is a disease but no dysfunction. Stage 2 is dysfunction—there is systolic or diastolic dysfunction or both, but the patient has never had symptoms. Stage 3 is chronic heart failure—cardiomyopathy with dysfunction due to the cardiomyopathy and patient has had symptoms of heart failure. Stage 4 is end-stage heart failure (same as New York Heart Association Class 4).

- **Left ventricular diastolic dysfunction Stages I–III:** Patients with no symptoms, only findings on echo, are not chronic heart failure patients. Stages II and III have symptoms.

Documentation needs

- With the documentation of CHF, clarify whether you are discussing right heart failure or left heart failure. If left heart failure, clarify whether this represents an acute or chronic state or both (provide BNP level).

- Document the etiology of the cardiomyopathy (hypertensive heart disease, ischemic heart disease, valvular and which valve[s], viral, alcoholic, etc.).

- Document known results of cardiac function studies and state whether they reflect failure due to left ventricular systolic dysfunction, left ventricular diastolic dysfunction, or both.

- Clarify the patient's heart failure status (due to chronic left ventricular systolic or diastolic dysfunction) and whether the current episode reflects acute decompensation (e.g., "Patient with chronic diastolic failure due to hypertensive heart disease with acute systolic decompensation due to non-Q wave MI").

- Document whether the patient had an acute MI within eight weeks of this episode and whether the acute MI was the cause of this episode of decompensation. (Will change to four weeks with ICD-10.)

- Name/document the relationship if this is a patient with chronic renal failure (CRF) and if volume overload or noncardiac pulmonary edema led to the decompensation of CHF.

Hyperglycemia

Elevated blood sugar can occur in many conditions and does *not* automatically mean that the patient has diabetes or that the patient with known diabetes has "uncontrolled" diabetes. Coverage with insulin around the time of illness or surgery does not signify "uncontrolled diabetes."

Patients with diabetes can develop elevated blood sugar with use of steroids for another condition, such as COPD or allergy, with infection, and with stress. Uncontrolled diabetes usually implies long-term lack of control and can be measured with glycosylated hemoglobin, or hemoglobin A1C, over 7.0 or difficulty in maintaining a job, good grades in school, or psychological balance over a long period of time.

Diabetes mellitus has four major classifications:

- **Type 1**—patient born with or acquired inability to produce insulin and cannot live without insulin

- **Type 2**—acquired resistance to effects of insulin; may be diet controlled, on oral hypoglycemics, or may take insulin for added control

- **Secondary causes of diabetes**—due to genetic disorder or poisoning of the islet cells or long-term use of steroids or after pancreatic surgery (see *http://www.hcpro.com/HIM-223721-147/Go-back-to-the-source-when-coding-secondary-diabetes.html*)

- **Gestational diabetes**—diabetes during pregnancy that resolves after delivery

Diabetic ketoacidosis or diabetic hyperosmolar coma can occur with extremely high levels of sugar.

Diabetes can have adverse effects on target organs:

- Diabetic retinopathy

- Diabetic nephropathy

- Diabetic autonomic neuropathy (with gastroparesis or Charcot foot or skin ulcer)

- Diabetic dermopathy—discolorations without serious side effects

- Diabetic microvascular disease—can lead to gangrene of distal extremities, cerebral ischemia, heart ischemic

Documentation needs

- Document whether the patient has diabetes. Define when it is uncontrolled. Although hemoglobin A1C determination may be helpful, your clinical impression is just as important.

- Document whether the patient has type 1 (i.e., does not make insulin), type 2 (i.e., is resistant to insulin), or other secondary cause of diabetes. If this patient has adult-onset diabetes and is taking insulin, document "type 2, taking insulin," and not "insulin dependent" (avoid using the terms IDDM and NIDDM).

- Name the infectious source if this episode was precipitated by an infection. If this incident represents sepsis from a source, name/document it as "sepsis due to _____." If related to an indwelling device (e.g., cardiac valve, Foley catheter, vascular access device), name that device as the source.

- Document whether the patient has other manifestations of diabetes (e.g., gastroparesis, diabetic renal failure, blindness, or neuropathy).

- Name/document the reason for hyperglycemia (e.g., steroid therapy, other endocrine dysfunction) if this patient is not diabetic.

Low Anterior Resection

Cancers of the large intestine are classified, for the purposes of the tumor registry and other tracking, by the location of the cancer in the bowel. Treatment of these cancers is similarly classified by the portion of the intestine removed. Surgeons use CPT codes to bill for their procedures. For most of the surgeries performed, they use one particular CPT code, which reads "partial resection of colon with low pelvic anastomosis." This definition may lead some doctors astray in describing the operation they performed from the perspective of ICD-9-CM coding.

Low anterior resection is an operation designed for resection of a cancer in the midportion of the rectum with end-to-end anastomosis. If end-to-end anastomosis is impossible for these rectal cancers, an abdominoperineal resection is the alternative.

Other colon resections for colon cancers include right hemicolectomy, left hemicolectomy, sigmoidectomy, total abdominal colectomy, and other resections (e.g., resection of the transverse colon for cancers located in the midportion of the transverse colon).

Other pathologic conditions may lead to similar operative procedures, such as diverticulitis, multiple polyposis, and ulcerative colitis. For proper ICD-9-CM coding, you need the portion of the intestine that the pathologic condition is located in, the name of that pathologic condition, and the portion of the large intestine actually removed.

Documentation needs

- Define and document in the medical record whether the disease process originated in the sigmoid colon, originated in the rectum, or was specified at the rectosigmoid junction.

- Clarify/document whether the disease was of the sigmoid colon or rectum in resections for diverticular disease.

- Specify/document which part of the bowel was resected (e.g., sigmoidectomy, rectal resection) if there is cancer or a premalignant lesion. The tumor board collects data based on location of the malignancy and the part of bowel removed even though you bill by resection with or without colostomy or with low pelvic anastomosis. Specifying/documenting this information makes the data more valuable.

Note: In cases of anemia due to chronic blood loss from the lesion (diverticular bleed or malignant lesion bleed), specify/document that the anemia was due to chronic blood loss from the lesion.

Malignancies

Neoplasms, or tumors, may involve almost any tissue. They may be **benign, malignant,** or **indeterminant** by pathologic examination. The malignancies may be localized to a spot in an organ, may have spread from the original spot but are still within the organ, may have spread to other tissues adjacent to and outside of the organ, or may have metastasized to regional lymph nodes or through the bloodstream to other organs, such as the liver, lungs, or brain.

The following is required for proper determination of the current status of the patient:

- The name of the primary tumor if the primary tumor is present
- Whether it is benign or malignant
- Whether there is spread to other tissues regionally
- Whether there is spread to lymph nodes
- Whether there is spread to other organs and which specific organs
- If the primary has been removed and the patient is admitted for surgery for metastatic disease, each organ to which metastatic

disease is identified must be named (principal diagnosis is the metastatic site)

- Whether the patient is admitted for workup and determination of the original diagnosis or admitted for radiotherapy or chemotherapy with the diagnosis having already been made

- Whether the patient is admitted only for treatment of a manifestation of the tumor, such as anemia (the anemia would be the principal diagnosis)

- Whether the patient is admitted for pain control with no treatment directed at the cancer (the cancer would be the principal diagnosis)

- Whether the patient is converted to hospice care or Comfort Measures Only

- Whether the patient is admitted with terminal cancer and no diagnosis has been made pathologically but all tests signify that it is undoubtedly cancer; if the physician is sure that is the problem, it is coded as though the cancer diagnosis has been made

Documentation needs

- Identify/document the primary source of the malignancy and whether that primary source is still being treated or has been treated and is no longer present. Do not use the term "history of" if the malignancy is still present. Only use this term if the primary source is totally gone.

- Identify/document whether there is a recurrence at the same site or a reappearance at a different site (i.e., metastasis—and to what site).

- Clarify/document the organ of reappearance versus the organ of origin ("lung met" could be interpreted as either metastasis of testicular cancer to the lung or metastasis of lung cancer to the brain, unless you are specific).

- Clarify in your documentation whether current symptoms are related to direct invasion of the malignancy, related to the pressure effect, or totally unrelated to the presence of the malignancy.

- Document a malignancy as a malignancy if a scan or x-ray confirms it. "Mass" is not "cancer." "Tumor" is not "cancer." You do not need biopsy confirmation to call it a cancer if you truly believe it is a malignancy.

- In documentation of leukemias, clarify whether this visit involves leukemia in remission, leukemia cured, or leukemia never having (yet) achieved remission. "History of" does not tell the story.

Malnutrition

Background

Malnutrition has adverse effects on the body's ability to defend itself against invading microorganisms, to heal after surgery or trauma, and to maintain homeostasis during any hospital intervention.

Malnutrition can be represented by inadequate intake of proteins, fats, and sugars as well as vitamins, minerals, and other substances that the body requires to perform daily functions. Many of the conditions caused by the lack of vitamin and mineral intake have their own specific names (e.g., iron deficiency anemia, scurvy, pellagra), so they will not be further discussed in this area.

Many disease states have malnutrition inherent in them as a risk factor, and preventive treatments are often in place to prevent malnutrition, such as with short gut syndrome, where a patient may be on nutritional supplements or intravenous hyperalimentation in order to maintain good nutritional status. Most patients with cirrhosis, terminal malignancies, renal failure, or who are on high-powered antimetabolites and chemotherapeutic drugs (as in cancer therapy) are constantly malnourished.

For tracking purposes, malnutrition has been stratified into mild, moderate, and severe. When protein stores are severely depleted, whether acutely or chronically, protein energy malnutrition (formerly called protein calorie malnutrition) occurs.

Patients who are severely protein depleted may be edematous because of the lack of protein to maintain intravascular oncotic pressure, but may appear healthy. Other patients may look cachectic or wasted. It is important to define and stratify the level of malnutrition in these patients. The terms "kwashiorkor" and "marasmus" are not normally used in the United States; however, these patients also have protein malnutrition. These specific terms are not needed to determine that a patient has protein calorie malnutrition or to stratify the level as mild, moderate, or severe. The proper ICD code assignment is for "other severe protein calorie malnutrition."

Many screening tools exist for determination of this severity—they are often called **subjective global assessments** of nutrition. The physician's ability to look at a patient and the patient's history may be all that is necessary to determine that a patient is severely malnourished.

Levels of protein alone, of albumin alone, or of prealbumin are inadequate to determine the presence, much less the level, of malnutrition. Addition of such evaluations as patient's body mass index (BMI) or percentage of loss in body weight (specifically *not* loss in water weight, as can happen with diuretics, removal of ascites, or delivery of a baby) can make a difference. Most authorities will recognize that unplanned loss of body mass under 10% represents mild malnutrition, between 10% and 20% is consistent with moderate malnutrition, and over 20% implies severe malnutrition.

Malnutrition evaluation in children has specific guidelines as related to expected levels of growth and development. Several methodologies are utilized that compare weight-to-height ratios, weight-for-age ratios, BMI, and deviation from expected and other techniques.

Malnutrition in the newborn is often related to problems with the mother and her nutritional habits. Review of the dietary notes can be helpful.

In addition to the presence of malnutrition stratified by severity, it is clinically pertinent to identify the cause of the malnutrition:

- Acute malnutrition due to complex trauma or extensive surgery.

- Acute malnutrition due to acute disease such as acute ischemic bowel disease, clostridia enterocolitis, necrotizing pancreatitis, sepsis.

- Chronic malnutrition due to chronic disease such as Crohn's disease, short bowel syndrome, chronic ischemic bowel disease, cancer, etc.

- Chronic malnutrition due to child or elder abuse by not feeding the person.

- Chronic malnutrition due to psychological disorder such as bulimia, other psychological disease.

- A morbidly obese person can be severely malnourished. Malnutrition should also be considered in psychological disturbances, including binging/purging manifestations, as can happen with bulimia.

Documentation needs

- It has been identified that your patient has lost ____ pounds over the past ____ months. This translates to a ____% loss in body mass.

- Your patient's BMI has been identified as ____% (under 17%) and there is an order for dietary supplementation using _____. Identification of malnourished state and stratifying its severity is important in determining increased risk to healing.

- Please help us identify whether the patient's nutritional status is depleted and stratify the level of malnutrition (mild, moderate, severe), if appropriate. (Provide the documented clinical evidence to support the need for this question.)

Note: The terms **cachexia** or **wasted appearance** are identified by most physicians at the time of admission. Identification of the cause of this appearance may be beneficial in stratifying the patient's risk.

Obesity

Obesity poses a serious risk to a satisfactory outcome in the hospital. In fact, physical and metabolic aspects of the obese patient can lead to the need for hospitalization. Obese patients have a higher risk of complications from anesthesia and surgery, and concomitant malnutrition that can occur in these patients can hinder resistance to infection.

Obesity is stratified grossly as obese and **morbidly obese,** with the latter being defined as 100 pounds over ideal body weight, or a BMI of 40 or above. Most morbidly obese patients will develop secondary diseases such as the following:

- Type 2 diabetes

- Hypertension with left ventricular strain causing left ventricular hypertrophy and diastolic dysfunction

- Gastroesophageal reflux

- Cellulitis under the folds of the pannus or under the arms

- Osteoarthrosis of the joints of the leg leading to need for joint replacement surgery

People living with a large abdominal size for long periods of time may develop **obesity hypoventilation syndrome (Pickwickian syndrome),** with pressure from the abdomen resulting in regurgitation at night that leads to the following:

- Sleep apnea

- Restriction of the movement of the diaphragm with respiration leading to secondary pulmonary hypertension from the restrictive lung disease, which leads to the following:

    - Right heart strain

- Chronic cor pulmonale, which leads to the following:

    - Increased venous pressure starting in the right atrium, which leads to the following: Chronic passive congestion of the liver

    - Cardiac cirrhosis

    - Ascites

    - Deep venous disease in the legs

    - Secondary hypercoagulable state

    - Edema of the legs with cellulitis

All of these should be documented when they exist, as they may individually or as a group lead to in-hospital morbidity and mortality.

Documentation needs

- Clarify/document whether your patient identified as overweight is, indeed, obese. BMI has been determined to be _____.

- Identify/document patients who are morbidly obese as this carries a significant increase in morbidity and mortality outcomes for hospitalization.

- Identification of patients with morbid obesity is important in order to track the secondary conditions associated with morbid obesity (e.g., diabetes, hypertension, gastroesophageal reflux, osteoarthrosis of hips and knees).

- Identification of patients with obesity hypoventilation syndrome is important because of the added risk of morbidity and mortality associated with this condition (e.g., restrictive lung disease, cor pulmonale, congestive liver disease, secondary hypercoagulable state). Identify each of the problems your patient demonstrates from obesity hypoventilation syndrome.

Pneumonia

Pneumonias are classified by the organism causing the infection, if known, or by three other entities: aspiration pneumonitis (which includes aspiration pneumonia), **empyema** (infected pleural effusion or pyothorax), and **lung abscess.**

Loeffler's syndrome, also known as **eosinophilic pneumonia,** is an allergic phenomenon. **Hypostatic pneumonia** is a postmortem finding—no patients are admitted for treatment of hypostatic pneumonia. The term was originated to depict settling of blood in the lungs from long-term (months to years) immobility and is found in the end stages of terminal illness. Do *not* encourage use of this term.

Pneumonitis is a chemical inflammation of the lungs that can be caused by aspiration of gastric acid or other toxic chemicals. It can be followed by true pneumonia because of the setting up of irritated areas in the lung that will be prone to secondary infection.

Aspiration pneumonitis, aspiration pneumonia, and **aspiration bronchitis** are defined, for the purposes of ICD-9-CM coding, as related to aspiration of foodstuffs or gastric content that can lead to acute pulmonary edema and acute respiratory distress syndrome (ARDS) with acute respiratory failure, persistent coughing and wheezing, or an indolent infection in an elderly patient. It is not to be mistaken for the mode of transmission of bacteria into the lungs from a patient's mouth or through droplet transmission from another person.

Hospital core measures guidelines for pneumonia patients include administration of "appropriate antibiotics" within two hours of diagnosis. To that end, those patients at high risk of aspiration pneumonia or *Pseudomonas* pneumonia or any other identifiable organism through culture or history should have antibiotic regimens prepared for those organisms. The physician should evaluate all pneumonia admissions for these contingencies.

Pneumonia is a clinical diagnosis, and pneumonias can be diagnosed with normal chest x-rays if the clinical findings and physical examination convince the physician. If an initial thought of pneumonia is made in the emergency department but further notes regarding the patient no longer mention pneumonia, clarify whether it was ruled out as a valid diagnosis.

Ventilator-associated pneumonia is pneumonia that develops after a patient has been on a ventilator for a period of time; it does not identify a patient admitted with pneumonia who requires a ventilator for acute respiratory failure.

Documentation needs

- Evaluate the patient's risk of aspiration as the cause of the pneumonia from the perspectives of debilitating GERD, alcoholism, bed-ridden status, pharyngeal dysfunction, etc. Document whether you believe that this is a case of aspiration pneumonia or aspiration pneumonitis.

- Clarify/document whether the "infiltrate" identified in your notes from the chest x-ray likely represents pneumonia, CHF, chronic lung disease, ARDS, Loeffler's syndrome, atelectasis, lung cancer, etc.

- Document in the medical record whether you are using antibiotics to treat specific organisms that you believe are the likely cause of pneumonia (e.g., *Klebsiella, Pseudomonas, Streptococcus,* Methicillin-resistant *Staphylococcus aureus,* Methicillin-sensitive *Staphylococcus aureus,* aerobic Gram negative rods) even in the absence of positive sputum culture.

- Identify/document patients admitted with pneumonia that started with specific influenza virus infections (e.g., novel swine influenza, avian influenza) and distinguish them from a patient who has pneumonia and an incidental positive test for specific influenza viruses, unrelated to the pneumonia.

- *Example:* If you believe that this case represents pneumonia, despite a normal chest x-ray in a patient who is dehydrated or otherwise does not demonstrate an infiltrate, clarify it in the medical record.

Pulmonary Edema

Background

Fluid in the interstitial spaces in the lung or fluid in the alveoli can be interpreted as **pulmonary edema.** With severe shortness of breath, it is likely **acute pulmonary edema.** Chronic pulmonary edema is usually a manifestation of end-stage heart failure. Patients with acute pulmonary edema may present with acute respiratory failure.

Cardiac causes of acute pulmonary edema include:

- Exacerbation of left ventricular heart failure including with volume overload in ESRD patients who have chronic heart failure

- Acute MI, whether from coronary occlusion or demand MI

- Accelerated (or malignant) hypertension including the severe hypertension that may occur with thyrotoxicosis, pheochromocytoma, carcinoid syncrome, eclampsia

- Tachyarrhythmia (AF with RVR, supraventricular tachycardia, ventricular tachycardia)

- Takotsubo syndrome (stress cardiomyopathy or apical ballooning syndrome)

Noncardiac causes of acute pulmonary edema include:

- Pulmonary embolism (venous thrombi, fat or air embolism)

- Aspiration of gastric acid

- Aspiration of toxic fumes and vapors

- Sepsis (ARDS)

- Rapid decompression

- Drowning

- Volume overload in ESRD patients who do not have chronic heart failure

Documentation needs

- Was this an acute MI (including non-Q wave MI due to ventricular tachycardia, pulmonary embolism, or fat embolus)? If so, document it as the cause of the pulmonary edema.

- Was there chest trauma, rapid deceleration, sepsis, or ARDS? If so, document that as the cause of the pulmonary edema.

- Did the patient aspirate fumes, vapors, gastric acid, or food? If so, document it as the cause of the pulmonary edema.

- Is this volume overload related to renal failure with an otherwise stable heart? If so, document it as noncardiac pulmonary edema.

If this is an ESRD patient with heart failure due to volume overload, state so.

- *Example:* "Noncompliant patient missed dialysis two days ago, admitted now in volume overload causing exacerbation of chronic diastolic heart failure."

Renal Failure

As with other diseases, there are chronic changes to renal function as well as acute changes that can occur. **Acute renal failure** (or acute kidney injury) can be of varying severity, from various causes, and can lead to total resolution or residual deficit in renal functional capabilities.

CKD has a myriad of causes, with the most frequent in the United States being diabetes and hypertension. Decreases in renal function can progress very slowly or very rapidly. The National Kidney Foundation supports following a patient's GFR to determine whether there is change, and if there is decrease in function, taking measures to control the disease that has caused that decrease in function. If progress is rapid, the patient must be prepared for dialysis or transplantation, if clinically appropriate.

CKD is staged according to GFR using formulas that are designed for infants and children (Schwartz equation) and for adults up to age 83 (Fadem equation). There are five recognized stages of progressive severity, as shown in Figure 1.

Figure 1: Five stages/severity chart

Stage	Severity	GFR
1	Kidney damage with normal or raised GFR:	>90 ml/min/1.73m^2
2	Kidney damage with mild decrease in GFR:	60-90 ml/min/1.73m^2
3	Moderate decrease in GFR:	30-59 ml/min/1.73m^2
4	Severe decrease in GFR:	15-29 ml/min/1.73m^2
5	Kidney Failure GFR:	<15 ml/min/1.73m^2

Stage 5 is considered kidney failure and, depending on the clinical situation, may require dialysis. When a patient with Stage 4 or 5 CKD has been on chronic dialysis for three months, the patient is considered ESRD for billing purposes.

Acute renal failure can occur from many causes, the most common of which is severe dehydration. Due to toxicity from acetaminophen or from iodide dyes used for contrast radiography or aminoglycosides (gentamicin, tobramycin, amikacin), efforts must be made to avoid kidney injury when these drugs are given. Treatment of acute renal failure ranges from rehydration to acute need for dialysis.

Changes in creatinine level or urine output may define the three stages of acute renal failure (acute kidney injury [AKI]). A person who is dehydrated should not be identified as having suffered from acute renal failure until having been resuscitated for at least six hours. If creatinine levels return to predehydration level, the patient was merely dehydrated. Distinction must be made between elevated creatinine level due to hemoconcentration and AKI, which does not immediately respond to fluid challenge. (See Figure 2.)

Figure 2: AKI stages chart

AKI stage	Creatinine criteria	Urine output criteria
AKI stage I	Increase of serum creatinine by >/= 0.3 mg/dl (>/= 26.4 umol/L) or increase to >/= 150% – 200% from baseline	Urine output < 0.5 ml/kg/hour for > 6 hours
AKI stage II	Increase of serum creatinine to > 200% – 300% from baseline	Urine output < 0.5 ml/kg/hour for > 12 hours
AKI stage III	Increase of serum creatinine to > 300% from baseline or (>/= 354 ?mol/L) after a rise of at least 44 umol/L or treatment with renal replacement therapy	Urine output < 0.3 ml/kg/hour for > 24 hours or anuria for 12 hour

Documentation needs

- Recognize that acute renal failure is not the same as acute renal insufficiency. If the creatinine rises 0.3 mg higher than the patient's normal level, this is consistent with failure or AKI. If due to dehydration and the patient's creatinine returns to baseline within six hours, it was not AKI.

- Document the cause of the acute renal failure (e.g., severe dehydration, acute tubular necrosis, sepsis, rhabdomyolysis, obstruction).

- Determine the stage of CKD in all patients with previously documented chronic renal insufficiency (CRI) or chronic renal failure (CRF). Using the stages will determine severity of illness. Although CRI or CRF is now useless for that determination, you can still use ESRD when the patient has been on chronic dialysis (three months).

- Use the GFR calculator (MDRD or Cockroft, or Schwartz formula for children and infants) to determine GFR and convert it to the appropriate CKD stage. Document it in inpatient or outpatient medical records. The complexity of medical decision-making also depends on this information.

Note: When a patient has CKD, regardless of stage, document the cause of the renal disease (e.g., HTN, diabetes, chronic pyelonephritis, lupus nephritis, myeloma).

Respiratory Failure

Background

Delivery of oxygen to the body and elimination of carbon dioxide is the goal of respiration. When anything happens that significantly impairs the processes to meet that goal, the patient is in respiratory failure (unless the patient is purposely anesthetized or sedated and being maintained on a ventilator to avoid respiratory failure).

Many conditions can block delivery of oxygen or impede the clearance of carbon dioxide or both. **Hypoxemic respiratory failure** is referred to as **type 1 respiratory failure; ventilatory failure** or **hypercapnic respiratory failure** is referred to as **type 2.**

Chronic

Patients may be in a chronic state of respiratory failure due to musculoskeletal diseases (polio or cervical spine injury with paralysis of respiratory muscles), alveolar damage (e.g., pulmonary fibrosis, emphysema) or obstructive airways (e.g., COPD, bronchiectasis, cystic fibrosis). These patients will demonstrate hypoxemia with PaO_2 under 55 on room air or compensated respiratory acidosis with hypercapnia with either pH = 7.4 and pCO_2 over 50 or HCO_3 on basic metabolic panel over 30 (in the absence of other acid-base imbalance).

Acute

Patients may present with acute respiratory failure due to many causes, whether musculoskeletal in origin, as with acute spinal injury; viral infections that lead to paralysis (e.g., Guillain-Barre syndrome); overdoses of narcotic or illicit drugs; severe hypoxemia due to pulmonary embolism (whether venous, fat, or air in origin); damage to the lung tissue, as with inhalation of acid, alkaline fumes, or gastric acid; loss of functional lung tissue, as in severe atelectasis; pneumothorax or pleural effusion; ARDS from numerous possible causes; obstruction from acute exacerbations of COPD from pneumonia or bronchitis or unknown cause; exacerbations of cystic fibrosis; or a foreign body.

These patients will have acute distress in breathing, often using accessory muscles of respiration (neck muscles, abdominal breathing), breathing rapidly (over 28 breaths per minute), unable to speak more than two-word sentences, or exhibiting peripheral cyanosis. They may respond rapidly to interventional drugs or other specific treatments and, by the time they get to the nursing unit, no longer demonstrate any of these symptoms—but the circumstances of admission certainly included acute respiratory failure.

What is not acute respiratory failure

Some patients will be intubated and placed on a ventilator for protective reasons when there is not (yet) acute respiratory failure, as with patients who have had a significant stroke or who have laryngeal angioedema due to allergic reaction. Patients electively being maintained on a ventilator overnight only to be weaned the next day when there is a full team available do not have acute respiratory failure.

Documentation needs

- Document in the medical record whether you believe that the patient has respiratory failure in addition to any other diagnoses in this case.

- Document whether the respiratory failure is acute, chronic, or with acute decompensation (acute-on-chronic).

- Name/document the basic disease causing the respiratory failure. Clarify the acute process on top of a chronic disease (e.g., acute respiratory failure due to pneumonia in a patient with chronic respiratory failure from multiple sclerosis).

- Document clinical signs, symptoms, and any laboratory findings to support the diagnosis of acute respiratory failure, when present.

- Document in the progress notes and discharge summary if the patient had acute respiratory failure upon admission and it resolved.

Seizures

There are several conditions where patients may have seizure activity but they do not represent epilepsy. It is important to differentiate these from epilepsy as a person's job may depend on such a distinction.

Epilepsy is a condition of recurrent seizures of varying magnitude resulting from the generation of aberrant electrical impulses in the brain. It cannot be cured but may respond to medications or, in some cases, surgical intervention.

Types identified include **petit mal** (may present as stopping in mid-sentence, smacking lips, blinking eyes rapidly, then resolves); **grand mal** (often tonic-clonic movements of extremities or the whole body); **Jacksonian seizures** (marching of tonic activity from one area to another); or **partial seizures,** which may be **simple** (without loss of consciousness, lasting 90 seconds or less, with either abnormal sensations or some jerking), or **complex** (with loss of consciousness, lasting one to two minutes—differentiated from petit mal by the length of the event).

Most cases of epilepsy (70%–75%) do not have a significant historical event that one can point to and are considered idiopathic. Patients may develop seizure activity during infections of the brain or as a result of scarring in the brain after an infection, such as with encephalitis, during strokes or as a late effect of strokes because of the healing process of the stroke, with brain neoplasms, or after removal of brain neoplasms, again because of scarring. When a seizure occurs during the acute event, it is a seizure due to that condition and is not (yet) epilepsy. However, when a patient develops recurring seizures (more than two) linked to these delayed circumstances, this is hallmark for a diagnosis of epilepsy.

Repeated grand mal seizure activity without significant resolution between seizures is called **status epilepticus;** this can lead to respiratory failure.

Seizures of epilepsy may be heralded by an aura that it is coming again and, when of the grand mal variety, may be associated with loss of bowel or bladder function and may be followed by loss of consciousness or amnesia for the event (postictal state).

Mostly in children, fevers can cause seizure called **febrile convulsion.** This is not epilepsy. Simple febrile seizures are generalized convulsions that last less than 15 minutes and do not recur within 24 hours. Complex febrile seizures can be generalized or focal and often last longer than the simple variety, but do recur within 24 hours. They are often associated with more serious infections than the usual viral illnesses of children. These seizures may not occur when the temperature is highest and may be the first sign that a viral infection has started.

Seizures can result from lesions in the temporal lobe of the brain, and these may be amenable to surgery if routine antiepileptic medications are not effective.

Documentation needs

- Document clearly whether you believe that the patient had a seizure (postictal state) or name another cause of alteration of consciousness.

- Document the relationship between other existing diseases (e.g., recent or old stroke, recent or old head trauma, brain tumor, febrile convulsion, drug overdose, alcoholism, diabetes out of control, viral or other infection, sepsis) and the seizure.

- Clearly state/document whether you determine that a known seizure patient aspirated at the time of the seizure event and when the respiratory problem prompted admission.

- State/document whether you believe that the patient has epilepsy to differentiate from other causes of seizure. Name the type (e.g., simple or complex partial epilepsy, grand mal, petit mal).

- State/document whether this event was initially thought to be a seizure and you determined that it was not a seizure.

Sepsis

Background

Sepsis is a series of chemical and biologic changes in response to an infection that may lead to progressive organ dysfunction and death if not countered by the body's defenses or treated with antibiotics, maintenance of failing organs, and sometimes surgery.

Bacteremia implies the presence of bacteria in the bloodstream, although not necessarily due to an infection. Bacteremia may exist along with sepsis or it may be a transient event caused by invasion of the bloodstream from a procedure that led to opening of the bloodstream to a source of infection. This occurs with dental cleanings, which is why patients with heart valve disease receive prophylactic antibiotics for every trip to the dentist, or why patients undergoing transrectal prostate biopsies receive a shot of prophylactic gentamicin or other antibiotic. Currently, infectious disease specialists believe that "bacteremia" is a better term for "septicemia due to bacteria," "viremia" is a better term for "septicemia due to viruses," and "fungemia" is a better term for "septicemia due to fungi." However, reflection of severity of illness is best illustrated with "septicemia due to."

Septicemia is infection of the bloodstream. Signs and symptoms of septicemia include shaking chills, rigors, temperature spikes, and significantly elevated white blood cell count. It also may coexist with sepsis. With the adoption of ICD-10, there will no longer be a designation for "septicemia;" bacteremia or bacterial sepsis will be preferred.

A **contaminant** implies that a blood sample was drawn without proper aseptic technique. This permitted growth of an organism on a culture plate but no infection exists due to that organism.

Colonization implies presence of bacteria in a body orifice or cavity without infection. This often occurs with patients who have indwelling urinary catheters. A positive urine culture in an asymptomatic patient likely represents colonization. Bacteria often colonize tracheostomy stomas and other openings. Patients with bronchiectasis or cystic fibrosis may have colonization with pseudomonas and not have an active infection.

Systemic inflammatory response syndrome is inherent with infections, and the term should not be used to imply "sepsis" when sepsis does not exist. Document noninfectious sources of systemic inflammatory response syndrome, such as necrotizing pancreatitis, massive body burns, large pulmonary emboli, etc.

Documentation needs

- Document in the medical record the source of the infection, if known.

- Document in the medical record the patient's signs and symptoms of sepsis.

- Document the presence of organ failure (e.g., acute renal failure, septic shock, acute respiratory failure, hepatic failure, critical care myopathy, or metabolic encephalopathy related to sepsis).

- Document whether positive blood cultures are clinically significant or represent contaminants. Remember, absence of positive blood culture does not preclude the diagnosis of sepsis.

- Document predisposing factors (e.g., immunocompromise, as in diabetes, steroid therapy, malnutrition, immunoglobulin deficiency, or chemotherapy).

- Document the likelihood of a relationship to implanted devices, such as heart valve (endocarditis), indwelling Foley catheter, vascular access device, etc.

- Avoid using terms such as "urosepsis" as a substitute for sepsis, as these words reflect a lower severity and acuity of your patient.

- Specify whether bacteremia is due to a septic condition in the body or is transient due to a procedure or unknown cause.

Stroke/Cerebrovascular Accident

Background

Stroke implies an acute brain event that leads to brain cellular death (infarction) or pressure from a hemorrhage against brain cells that prevents them from functioning properly. Strokes can range in severity from minimal with brief symptoms that resolve in minutes and was validated on a subsequent x-ray, to one with sudden loss of consciousness, paralysis, rapid cessation of breathing, and death.

There are two major types of stroke: ischemic and hemorrhagic.
An **ischemic** stroke may represent an embolism from the heart or from an ulcerated plaque of the carotid artery or a local occlusion of a vessel in the brain. A **hemorrhagic** stroke may be subarachnoid, intracerebral, or intraventricular. Ischemic strokes are identified by the artery involved in the occlusion, if known. Hemorrhagic strokes are identified by the portion of the brain involved with the hemorrhage.

Hemorrhagic strokes are grouped by the lobes of the brain involved; ischemic strokes are grouped by the major intracranial vessel occluded (when that is known). Both ischemic and hemorrhagic strokes benefit from documentation of which side of the brain was involved (right or left) and whether hemiparesis involved the patient's dominant or nondominant side.

A patient with a **subdural hemorrhage** may have spontaneous or traumatic hemorrhage after a fall and striking the head. For patients who fall a lot, it is sometimes difficult to know which came first.

A **TIA** is identified as a localizing, lateralizing neurologic deficit that lasts seconds to minutes, such as transient unilateral blindness (amaurosis fugax). It is caused by a platelet clot that briefly obstructs a vessel in the brain, then breaks apart and flow is immediately reestablished. Vertebrobasilar insufficiency occurs with transient occlusion of blood flow to the cerebellum or base of the brain and may manifest as a fall due to transient vertigo. Sometimes, tight collar syndrome can imitate a carotid TIA and subclavian steal syndrome can present as a vertebrobasilar attack.

If a CT scan on admission shows an infarct, it is probably an old infarct because, except for massive infarcts, one cannot detect ischemic strokes on CT. CT is performed to demonstrate whether a stroke is hemorrhagic.

Enzymes (such as tissue plasminogen activator) may be administered to a patient with an acute embolic or occlusive stroke if symptoms started within three hours of evaluation and the patient has no other bleeding problems. **Another option is mechanical embolism removal in cerebral ischemia,** which percutaneously removes a clot after embolism if caught within a few hours. Patients admitted with a stroke may have carotid narrowing (carotid stenosis) seen on flow studies. These are not to be construed as causative of the stroke unless the physician makes the link. Often, this is an incidental finding.

Documentation needs

- Document whether you determine that the patient had a hemorrhagic stroke (e.g., intracerebral hemorrhage, subarachnoid hemorrhage; name the portion of the brain involved) or had an occlusive or embolic cerebral infarction (name the vessel involved, if known).

- If you diagnose cerebral infarction, document whether it was due to primary intracerebral occlusion (and name the artery, if possible), carotid disease with embolism from an ulcerated plaque, or cardioembolic stroke.

- Document whether the patient had an evolving stroke that was aborted by enzyme or anticoagulant therapy.

- Document whether the study revealed carotid artery disease as the cause of the patient's current symptoms, and explain whether this hospitalization was because of current cerebral infarction (true stroke) or noninfarction cerebral embolism (TIA).

- Avoid using terms such as reversible ischemic neurological deficit, cerebrovascular accident, or only "stroke" as these may be misconstrued and lead to a code that does not represent the true condition.

- Report/document when the patient has clinical signs of increased intracranial pressure, brain shift, herniation (side to side of foramen magnum), spastic or flaccid quadriplegia, and coma. "Unresponsiveness" does not imply coma when that condition exists.

- When the family agrees to cease active treatment and let the patient die comfortably, Comfort Measures Only is a preferable term to use to indicate withdrawal of life support or that no further care will be administered, rather than the term DNR, which implies all treatment for all conditions will be undertaken up to a designated point.

Symptoms

Generally, patients are seen in the emergency department or the physician's office with some symptoms. After workup, a diagnosis or several diagnoses may come to light as having caused the symptoms. For capturing clinical data and for billing purposes, the symptoms are preferred to justify studies done. In the hospital, the diagnoses after workup are preferable, and the link of the diagnoses to those presenting symptoms is paramount to be sure that the proper sequencing of codes takes place.

When a patient is admitted for signs and symptoms and the diagnosis is never established, what you believe to be the cause takes precedence. Sometimes there is no way to determine the cause, so the sign or symptom becomes the principal diagnosis.

When signs and symptoms of an adverse effect of a prescription drug occur, the sign or symptom will be the principal diagnosis.

Documentation needs

- Document distinctly the relationship between signs and symptoms on admission and the diagnoses determined after workup.

- If a symptom may be due to either of two (or more) diagnoses that you have established, state/document this information distinctly.

- If a patient's symptoms could be due to several diseases, none of which you are sure the patient has, state/document so distinctly.

- Document the diagnosis that you believe exists whenever you order studies or treatments while the patient is in the hospital.

Note: For cardiac arrest or cardiorespiratory arrest, document the most likely cause of the event (e.g., acute MI, Takotsubo syndrome, ventricular tachycardia/fibrillation, stroke, sepsis with shock). If you cannot determine the cause, that is fine.

Syncope

Fainting is usually due to decreased blood flow to the brain, whether it be cardiogenic in origin or neurogenic. Certain historical events point to a likely cause of syncope or near syncope.

This must be differentiated from other clinical conditions, such as a fall from tripping or a history of repeated falls due to normal pressure hydrocephalus, muscular weakness due to stroke or as a late effect of a previous stroke, TIAs (especially posterior circulation of the brain), malnutrition with weakness, brain tumors, subarachnoid bleeds, or other strokes.

Common causes of **cardiogenic syncope** include bradycardia, tachycardia with reduced diastolic filling of the heart, symptomatic aortic stenosis (including hypertrophic obstructive cardiomyopathy), venous pooling as from tight belt syndrome, hypovolemia as can occur with severe dehydration, or massive hemorrhagic events (e.g., GI bleed, menorrhagia, ruptured aneurysm).

Neurogenic syncope includes vasovagal responses as from seeing something horrifying, rapid emptying of the bowels or bladder (called postmicturition syncope), adverse effect of beta blockers, primary autonomic nerve dysfunction, diabetic neuropathy, etc.

The clinician must rule out acute MI, stroke, and sepsis first.

Orthostatic vital signs, or increase in heart rate and drop in blood pressure when changing from supine to sitting or sitting to standing, is *not* the same as the disease **orthostatic hypotension.** Orthostatic drop in blood pressure with testing can be a clinical sign of a vast number of diseases, including most of those previously mentioned. True orthostatic hypotension usually represents adrenal insufficiency or primary autonomic neuropathy. Look for a disease from the previous paragraphs to explain the syncope.

Documentation needs

- Did the patient have an identifiable event, such as postmicturition syncope, cough-related syncope, frightening event, or sudden positional change? If so, name that in the medical record as the cause of the syncope.

- Was there causative dehydration, arrhythmia, or drug-drug interaction? If so, name/document the cause.

- Did the patient trip and fall? If so, document that in the medical record rather than calling it syncope when it wasn't.

- Did the patient have an acute MI, stroke, or sepsis? If so, name/document the condition as the cause of the syncopal episode.

- Did the patient have acute cerebrovascular insufficiency, or does he or she have signs of chronic cerebrovascular ischemia with an acute insufficiency event? If so, name/document it as the cause of the episode.

Trauma

Background

A great many visits to the emergency department are due to traumatic events. The appropriate designation of the damage to the body often depends on proper documentation that will lead to the code that tells the same story. Additionally, trauma teams are developed in hospitals to deal with multiple significant trauma. This particular group of patients is often tracked statistically within a group of cases that involve significant trauma to at least three body systems. Multiple broken bones constitute one body system, unless one of them is the skull and another includes at least six ribs.

Closed head injury can result in a laceration of the scalp or the brain, skull or facial bone fracture, or contusion or hemorrhage to the brain. It is inadequate to merely call it "closed head injury" unless there was no other damage identified. Specifying cerebral concussion, cerebral contusion, or cerebral hemorrhage has major implications for severity of a trauma case.

Specifying presence of unconsciousness or coma is important as well as identifying how long the patient was unconscious, if known, and whether the patient is expected to wake up. "Unresponsiveness" or assigning a Glasgow coma score to the patient does not translate into unconsciousness or coma.

Documentation needs

- Document the presence or history of cerebral concussion or cause of transient loss of consciousness, even if it was resolved by the time you saw the patient.

- Document whether the patient had hypovolemia or hypovolemic shock on admission in the presence of bleed or multiple bony fractures.

- Document the number of ribs fractured on each side.

- Document the fracture or dislocation of each bone and whether each was treated by stabilization or surgery or not treated at all. Do not identify fractures by joint involved.

- Document when a patient has pulmonary contusion with or without respiratory failure.

- Name the cause (e.g., fat embolism, pulmonary contusion, shock lung, aspiration pneumonitis, alcohol or drug abuse) if the patient has acute respiratory failure.

- Include all diagnoses established from admission of the trauma case through discharge.